RENEW HEALTH

Taking Control of Your Temple

Learn to Heal your Body, Lose Healthy Weight fast, and Improve your Spiritual, Mental and Physical well-being.

JACQUELINE AKUA OWUSU, M.D.

Forwarded by Teresa Ann Paul, R.N.

Renew Health: Taking Control of Your Temple

By Jacqueline Akua Owusu, M.D.

All Scripture quotations, unless otherwise noted, are from the King James Version of the Bible.

For permission requests, speaking inquiries, and bulk order purchase options, email *renewhealth001@gmail.com* or *talkwithdrj@gmail.com*.

ISBN: 978-0-9840161-4-3

Watch our **YouTube channel** for more content:
Dr Owusu Wellness & Skincare

Published by **OASIS Publishing**

Printed in the United States of America

Cover design and Interior Layout: Tudor Maier

Edited by: OASIS Publishing, Rena Bledsoe, Angelia Shepherd, & Teresa Ann Paul.

Table of Contents

DEDICATION

This book is dedicated to God, Almighty for giving me the revelation on how to eat right and engage in promoting a healthy lifestyle for myself and others. God, may you continue to use me and allow me to always be obedient to you for your glory! To God be the glory for the things He has done.

I would also like to dedicate this book to my two sons Matthew and Michael Bediako. Thank you for your constant support and love. Thank you for letting me know how much I am loved even when I am not in your presence. I dedicate you back to God our Father. May He who created you and knows your yesterday, today and tomorrow help you to discover your purpose in life and to fulfill it for His glory!

ACKNOWLEDGEMENTS

Writing this book could not have been possible without the knowledge obtained from the teachings of Dr. Robert Morse, N.D., and some intelligent, insightful and loyal doctors and individuals who are dedicated to plant based nutrition. I have obtained a wealth of knowledge on health and spirituality from Dr. Robert Morse's teachings and for that I am forever grateful.

I am also grateful to Ms. Alice Owusu, my supportive, sweet and reliable mother for always being there and encouraging me. To my best friend and sister Teresa Ann Paul, thank you for your loyalty, consistency, intelligence, beauty (inside and out) and always telling me the truth even if it is not what I am willing to hear. To my sister from another mother, Rena Bledsoe, thank you for your exceptional work ethics, for being a good friend, for editing this book and for loving me for who I am because the feeling is mutual.

I would like to thank Pastor Benjamin Whittaker, Pastor Myrtis Temple, Bishop Valeria Allen, Ms. Rosie Crumb (for your constant prayers, love and support), Mr. Jordan Ohene (for the one God chose to reveal this book through before there was even a book), Ms. Shirley Peavy, Ms. Diane Smith (my ride and die partner), my staff at Renew Health Clinic, members of Living Free Now Church and the countless number of people who have participated in and/or completed The Renew Health Transformation Program.

FORWARD

Irst and foremost, it is imperative to bestow The Most High God with honor, adoration and praise for using Dr. Jacqueline Owusu as a conduit to heal his people. This program is based upon biblical principles that The Most High God has instructed in his word as a template for our healing and well-being. The Renew Health Program is unique in that it takes a multifaceted approach on how to care for and maintain our entire existence. Your temple encapsulates your mind, body and soul. In order to maximize our potential and maintain a healthy, balanced existence we must adequately and appropriately care for our temple.

I was one of the first participants in this program and I can speak to its efficacy and how it has positively impacted me on all levels of my being. I personally have multiple chronic health conditions that have changed the quality of my life and at times limited my ability to function. Earlier this year I was thrust into a new health scare that along with my existing health issues propelled me into looking for other methods to alleviate or resolve my health problems.

As a healthcare worker myself I wanted to heal my body and not put a Band-Aid on my health problems, like in times past, by taking the conventional route of medication and other adjunct medical therapies. The Renew Health Program offered a physician guided, holistic approach to health and well-being. In two weeks, I started to see significant improvement and changes in my health. As a result of these changes, I have incorporated this program as a lifestyle and have developed a new way of thinking. This book has specific, detailed testimonials that will underscore the Program's validity. My testimony has been recorded on Dr. Owusu's YouTube channel (***Dr. Owusu Skincare & Wellness***).

The Pathophysiology explained in layman's terms in this book denotes how this program works. I highly encourage you to explore this nonconventional, holistic approach to caring for your temple. We can't continue to do the same things expecting different results. Thus, I challenge you to step outside the box, exercise your faith, utilize your determination and change the course of your life. This is the key to your success and living your best life. I believe in you as you become a new Renew Health Warrior. Congratulations!

Forward written by:
Teresa Ann Paul, RN
Leadership Consultant

Chapter One

The Purpose of this Book

And God said, Behold, I have given you every herb bearing seed, which is upon the face of all the earth, and every tree, in which is the fruit of a tree yielding seed; to you it shall be for meat. (Genesis 1:29).

Have you been diagnosed with Diabetes, Hypertension, High Cholesterol and/or other chronic diseases and you feel powerless about it? Do you gain weight easily and find it very difficult to lose weight? Then the principles in this book will help you. The Renew Health book is written for anyone who is experiencing health issues and those who want to take preventative measures to abort potential health problems. This book is not a science journal with complicated content or hard to understand random trials and research. This is a book based on evidence-based medicine, and the methods that were used have been tested on myself and on my patients. My patients and I continue to see positive results and significant improvement in our overall health and well-being. The outcomes were significant enough that I felt compelled to share this with anyone who wants to take a holistic approach to healing and well-being, especially for individuals where traditional methods have not yielded desired outcomes. This book is written in a simplistic manner such that it can be consumed, regurgitated, applied, and shared by anyone regardless of education, background, or experience. The language is intended to be understood by people of all walks of life in hopes that everyone will be able to understand how what we eat has a great impact on our health and on our lives.

Diseases do not have to plague our body and cause severe and disabling damage to our body. We have the power to take control of our health, to help decrease the risk of chronic diseases such as obesity, diabetes mellitus II, hypertension, hyperlipidemia, heart diseases, autoimmune disorders, gastrointestinal disorders, and a whole host of other acute and chronic problems. By choosing healthier foods, we can execute that power, seize control from lifelong poor habitual choices, and begin the journey to good physical well-being.

Many people leave the management of their health in the hands of their healthcare provider. Healthcare Providers receive formal education, on disease processes, to help navigate people's illnesses. Providers need commitment from their patients to educate themselves on their disease conditions. As patients educate themselves on their disease conditions, it allows Providers to develop better management of their care and it facilitates patient compliance. When patients are frustrated with the deterioration of their chronic diseases, so are Providers when their patients are not improving with their medications and treatment regimen. Safeguarding your health is a team effort. Medication is oftentimes paired with other regimes such as exercise and diet change to bring about the desired outcome. The Provider can prescribe and suggest these things, but it is up to us to implement them into our daily lives. Therefore, as the patient, we have the power to take control over our body and health. Getting knowledge, understanding the knowledge and using it properly is the key for success.

Poor dietary choices increase the risk of chronic diseases. In addition, there are also external factors (such as genetic factors, environmental factors, and socioeconomic factors), which further increases our risk. We may not be able to control all the external factors, but we can pay close attention to the healthy food choices we make in helping to prevent and decrease our risk of chronic diseases. Initially, incorporating healthy food choices such as fruits and vegetables into a healthy lifestyle can be overwhelming. By increasing the consumption of fruits and vegetables and consistently doing it daily, helps us to develop healthy habits.

We are creatures of habits and change is hard for us. There will be groups who may not agree with the concept of this health journey for wellness. This journey for wellness contradicts some aspects of formal education and cultural norms. One cannot force anyone to accept a message they are not ready to receive. However, I strongly believe that this book will communicate to individuals who are meant to embark upon a holistic, non-invasive approach to wellness that can combat or improve most illnesses. We have to change our mindset from the myths and beliefs that we have heard on the consumption of carbohydrates and proteins. In renewing our minds, we have to challenge ourselves by trying the program out and then deciding if what we have heard and accepted as truth is indeed accurate.

This is a **healing program**. Weight loss and vitality are benefits we reap as our body heals itself using the process of detoxification and regeneration in getting rid of toxins and renewing our cells. This health journey does work but it takes motivation, discipline, dedication, and consistency. These principles work just like it does with every important milestone in our lives. The goal is to get healthy and heal our bodies. As our body heals, this healing program can allow Providers to decrease or discontinue chronic medications. Therefore, I highly encourage you to work with your Healthcare Provider as you embark on this health journey. The effort you put in this program will be the health benefit that will be rewarded back to you.

Consuming fruits and vegetables for good health is not a new way of eating. The Father of Medicine, Hippocrates said: "Let thy Food be thy Medicine, and thy Medicine be thy Food." The right food choices can heal the body and decrease the risk of chronic diseases. Our body speaks to us every day. We have to be attuned to the message our body is giving us. For example, if we have pain and swelling, our body is communicating that we are acidic and/or inflamed. If we are experiencing acid reflux, we have to watch the food we are eating. If we are experiencing constipation and/or diarrhea, it boils down to the foods consumed. Our body sends us messages that something is not right and changes need to be made. We should view it as our body's way of communicating to us that something is wrong and not ignore the warning signs. We then have to work on finding the main cause of the problem and not just focus on treating the symptoms.

Incorporating fruits and vegetables into our life as the main staple of our diet is a lifestyle journey. We have to make sure that this is what we really want to do and make up our minds that we will follow through. Therefore, if we are not ready to start this healthy lifestyle change for the long haul, we should not begin this journey. The reason is that if we are not disciplined and/or consistent, we will reverse any positive changes to our health and body that we obtain. If the program becomes overwhelming, take it slow and make small changes daily. It is better to go slow and continue with the program than to abandon it because you could not stick to the plan. Small incremental changes lead to success in the long term. Know that the most challenging part of this program will be changing the mindset and the psychological ideas that we have concerning food.

Focus Point

What does your current diet consist of?

Write down what you currently eat in a day.

Chapter Two

How I Embarked on this Journey

The steps of a good man are ordered by the Lord: and he delighteth in his way. (Psalm 37:23)

I was never an overweight person growing up. I had an athletic build and loved working out while I was in college. I maintained my weight by working out. Over the years, my poor eating habits and the increased amount of dietary fats I was ingesting on a daily basis, took a toll on my body.

I am originally from Ghana, West Africa. I would eat a diet full of high starchy carbohydrates, high fats, high proteins with minimal fruits and vegetables. As a result, when I reached twenty-two years of age, the weight was steadily piling on.

I got married in 2002 and had my first child in 2003, while I was still in my Physician Residency training program. With the combination of stress, pregnancy, and poor eating habits, I gained weight to over two hundred pounds. Several months after my child was born, I hired a personal trainer who came to my home and worked out with me. She told me to eat a lean high protein diet, I lost some weight with this diet but was still considerably overweight . Three years after my first child, I had another child and I continued to struggle with my weight and poor eating habits, on and off, throughout the years.

Years passed and my husband of seventeen years left me and my two boys. I did not understand and I was devastated. I spiraled into depression and low self esteem. I continued to have an unhealthy relationship with food which eventually led me to develop Insulin Resistance. With insulin resistance, losing weight was even more difficult. I tried several diets, as well as juice and water fasting. I would lose some weight with some of the diets, others, I would not lose anything and once I stopped, I would gain all the weight back and more. I even paid for a gym membership and hired a personal trainer. I was so motivated and dedicated. I went to the gym at 3:30 in the morning, walked on the treadmill for one hour and trained with my personal trainer for 30 minutes. I worked out and trained for five days a week and I was consistent with this routine for six months until I hurt my knee. After I injured my knee, I had to take a break because it was so painful. In addition to my gym routine, I was placed on a meal plan which consisted of a moderate amount of protein, fat and minimal fruits and vegetables. During my recovery from my knee injury, I tried to maintain eating according to the meal plan I was given, however, I became discouraged because when I finally weighed myself, I weighed more than when I started. Therefore, I stopped going to the gym and stopped training. This discouragement and lack of motivation continued until I reached rock bottom. Most individuals judge heavy set people as not having willpower. That is not a correct assessment. Most of us have the willpower to embark on a diet, an exercise program, and/or a health journey but when we fail to see results or the goal is not achieved that is when disappointment sets in. Once the disappointment and/or discouragement sets in, we then revert back to making unhealthy food choices.

I finally admitted to myself that I had an unhealthy relationship with food and if I did not do something drastically, I was going to die prematurely and leave my young children. I did not know what to do, but I knew I had to find something that worked for me and was sustainable. I figured eating fruits and vegetables could not harm me. I had been exposed to some of Dr. Robert Morse's teaching on healing the body with fruits. So I started eating fruits (specifically apples) for one week. Six days after eating as many apples as I wanted, I weighed myself and I was down *thirteen* pounds. I was shocked.

The only reason I stopped eating the apples for a day or two was because I started experiencing intense itching and later developed rashes all over my body. I discovered what I was experiencing was severe detox symptoms. Days after learning that what I was experiencing was detoxification symptoms, I decided to continue eating the apples to heal my body. I ate apples for twenty-four days of that month and lost a total of twenty six (26) pounds. I was in awe. I repeated the consumption of fruits the next month but included a variety of fruits (all types of fruits) and lost another twenty (20) pounds the second month. The third month I lost eighteen (18) pounds and it finally dawned on me that I was on to something powerful. I watched as many of Dr. Morse's videos as I could to gain more awareness and knowledge as I continued to embark on my journey.

I studied all I could on food combination, fruit fasting and the healing of the body. I continued with my healing journey and introduced it to my patients who I was having a difficult time managing their chronic medical problems with medications. The patients who embarked on this journey also started seeing positive results with incredible weight loss, improvement in their blood pressure and diabetes. These improvements were significant enough that it required decreasing and discontinuing some of their chronic medications. This was such a revelation to me that I went into prayer about it. Shortly after praying about this, I was led to record my journey on Youtube to help others struggling with getting their body healed to gain vitality and wellness. I was also led to write this book called "Renew Health, Taking Control of Your Temple" and to develop a program called Renew Health Transformation Program. Interestingly, three years prior to this, I opened a private medical clinic called Renew Health Clinic, not knowing anything about the upcoming eating program or the book. The revelation of everything coming together in full circle is when I knew this was BIG and it was bigger than me and it was a purpose driven agenda by God. I am not saying that all you will eat on this program is fruits because the program has evolved with time to include a variety of plant-based foods (such as fruits, vegetables, legumes, nuts and seeds) for healing and wellness of the body.

From Disappointment to Purpose

God called me into ministry after I became a physician. When my ex-husband left me, my ministry was just beginning and I thought this has got to be a bad joke. I experienced shock, hurt, disappointment, rejection, anger, and betrayal. I cried to God many times. I did not understand, but I had to trust God. I did not know what to do. Gradually, God used other people to pull me out of depression, sorrow and low self-esteem and revealed the Bible to me. The Bible speaks of his goodness, his mercy, his love, his peace, his compassion and his forgiveness. Eventually, I became an ordained minister and God asked me to forgive my ex-husband. God reminded me of a book he encouraged me to write on Forgiveness many years before. I eventually forgave my ex-husband and wished him well. Forgiveness is not for the other person but it is for you. Even in those times, God was working things out for the good even though I could not see it at the time of the storm. I am who I am today because of that experience and many more. Looking back, I am grateful for the experiences that I had.

We are spirit, soul and body. What affects us emotionally, affects us mentally and physically causing us to make unhealthy choices including food as a source of comfort. To get a handle on our emotions, we need to tackle hurt, disappointment, rejection, shame, low self-esteem, and other negative emotions that are hindering us.

I want you to know that everyone has a purpose on this earth. God created you and placed you in your mother's womb to be born at this time on earth and he has a purpose for you. The problem is that a lot of people do not know their purpose and often wonder why they are on earth. The Bible states in Jeremiah 29:11-13: *"For I know the thoughts that I think toward you, saith the Lord, thoughts of peace, and not of evil, to give you an expected end. Then shall ye call upon me, and ye shall go and pray unto me, and I will hearken unto you. And ye shall seek me, and find me, when ye shall search for me with all your heart."*

God created us and put us on this earth with a plan and purpose. We do not know the plan and/or purpose God has for us. We discover our identity and the plan which is our purpose as we seek God and yield to his leadership and guidance. God is a big God with many resources that never dries out. God is our source and he uses many resources to sustain us. The resources, however, are not our source, so we should not focus and depend on the resources (like our jobs, marriages/relationships, children, business, and much more). Resources may dry out, the resource door can be closed, the job can be lost, and the business can crumble but our source (who is God) never changes.

Discovering our purpose is not overnight. It is a journey and it takes time. It takes a series of steps and experiences, with the help of God, to help us identify our purpose. The Bible states, *"The steps of a good man are ordered by the Lord: and he delighteth in his way."* (Psalm 37:23).

Pastor Rick Warren (Saddleback Church) wrote the book titled: "The Purpose Driven Life." In this book, Pastor Rick talks about an acronym spelled **S.H.A.P.E** which stands for:

S = **Spirituality (the spiritual gifts we get after receiving salvation)**

H = **Heart (what we are passionate about)**

A = **Abilities (the abilities we were born with)**

P = **Personality (our personality)**

E = **Experiences (our positive and negative experiences)**

All of these together "shape" us into who we are and what we are created for.

Therefore, whatever experiences we have had in life (whether negative or positive) is part of the discovering journey of who we are.

We all experience frustrating, hurtful, debilitating and disappointing situations in life. We may not understand why we are going through the negative experiences and it may not seem fair. Sometimes, we even think that God has forgotten us. Sometimes, we cannot even imagine that God would allow these bad times in our lives to happen (remember he does not cause it, he allows it to happen) for a greater good. Through these experiences we learn lessons which propel us to our destiny. Remember, our steps are ordered by the Lord and *"And we know that all things work together for good to them that love God, to them who are the called according to his purpose."* (Romans 8:28).

It does not feel good when we are going through bad times. When it all comes together, we see how it worked for the greater good and the purpose God has for us. We are who we are today because of the difficult times. It is with the difficult experiences that has propelled us to discover our destiny. God is always in the midst of the storm with us. The Scripture states, *"Be strong and of a good courage, fear not, nor be afraid of them: for the Lord thy God, he it is that doth go with thee; he will not fail thee, nor forsake thee."* (Deuteronomy 31:6).

Past or current experiences (such as rejection, disappointment, pain, betrayal, violation and more) are part of the ingredients in discovering and fulfilling our purpose. There is nothing we have gone through or going through that is a surprise to God. He says, *"Before I formed thee in the belly I knew thee; and before thou camest forth out of the womb I sanctified thee, and I ordained thee a prophet unto the nations."* (Jeremiah 1:5). Therefore nothing about our experiences yesterday, today or in the future surprises God. God does not allow anything to happen that he does not have a purpose for and at the right time, he will connect all the dots. We just have to trust God even when we do not understand. We must have faith and believe in Him.

When we are in a storm or a bad situation, we cannot see the hand of God. When we are in a storm or a situation, or when God is silent we feel like God has forgotten about us. However, rest reassured that God has not forgotten about us. He is working behind the scenes. Let us look back over our lives and see some of the areas in our situations that God helped us through. This same God is with us today and will help us through this situation as well.

I have love and compassion for people today because of what I suffered. How else would I be able to minister to divorced women or people going through difficult relationships if I had not experienced it myself? So, when we are going through storms, the God of comfort, will send people our way to comfort us, console us, support us, and even teach us. As we overcome the situation, God then orchestrates us to help others who have experienced the same thing we have experienced and overcome with his help. We do have a purpose that only we can fulfill, and it involves our life's experiences, the good, the bad, and the ugly.

Who can effectively minister to a person who has lost a child, a spouse, a family member, someone who has been sexually abused, someone neglected by their parents, someone who is homeless, or on drugs but someone who has experienced those very same things and has overcome? There is something in this lifetime that only you are ordained to do. We are special individuals to God. We have a personal purpose that God has given to each and everyone of us.

Looking back on my health and weight journey, no matter what I did, I could not lose weight but it was all part of God's plan in leading me to discover this healing journey. Although my medical degree gives me credibility, God is the one who orchestrated and ordered my steps in discovering and sustaining this health journey. It was in my struggle in dealing with Insulin Resistance and obesity that caused me to look for solutions for my problem. My search led me to discover renewing our health with plant-based foods and herbs, eventually leading to the writing of this book and the Renew Health program. The Renew Health Transformation Program (RHTP) has saved me and many others. Therefore, if God directed me to discover and understand a solution to my problem, he will answer your problems too. It may not be the answer you want but it will be the right answer.

We have to trust God even when we don't understand. Thanking him for the things he is putting together behind the scenes for our benefit. When we are making a cake, there are many ingredients that are put together. The *different ingredients* can be looked at as our many experiences in life. The *finished cake* can be looked at as our purpose. Know that God has not forgotten us, all of our steps have been ordered by God. All things work together for the good and at his appointed time God will place the right people in the right place at the right time in our lives. God is with us now and he has not forgotten about us or our situations.

How is trusting God with all that we are and committing our ways to Him associated with renewing our health? We are complicated but complete beings. We are spirit, soul and body. We have a mind; we have emotions; and we have a free will to make choices. Therefore, what affects our mind, emotions, and our body, also affects our choices, our health, and our overall well being. I pray we draw close to God to discover our purpose and to fulfill it for His glory.

Focus Point

What is your S.H.A.P.E?

Write down your S.H.A.P.E and pray to God to help you forgive those who have wronged you.

What is your Purpose in life? If you do not know, ask God to show you what it is.

Chapter Three:

How Foods Affect Our Body?

The consumption of unhealthy foods and improper food combinations can affect our body. It can cause acidosis, inflammation, unhealthy gut, many chronic diseases and much more. However, our body is a living conscious machine. No matter how sick our body has become, it can detoxify and regenerate itself if it is not too far gone. Our body can rebuild itself with wholesome, living foods like raw, fresh fruits and vegetables. Detoxification is the body's way of cleansing itself of toxins, mucus, and acidosis which has clogged and obstructed the body with the prolonged eating of unhealthy foods.

Acidosis

Animal proteins and dairy, when eaten routinely, increase the production of acid in our body making them known as high acid foods. A high acid diet increases the risk of type II diabetes, heart disease, kidney disease, inflammation and more. Dairy products and processed grains, when consumed and digested, act like glue in our tissues. This mucoid plaque is irritating, mucus forming, and inflammatory to our body. Animal flesh and processed foods also cause inflammation and contain deadly chemicals and heavy metals that are harmful to our body. Cooked and processed foods slow down the body's elimination of toxins. In most cases, toxic by-products of foods are stored and cause plaque in tissues. This toxicity does not allow the cells to breathe properly causing the cell to become hypoactive, and eventually losing its ability to function.

Many disease symptoms are nothing more than our body's effort to eliminate stored toxins. Some of our chronic diseases we face today took root while we are still in our mother's womb. Weakened genes from the food we eat are passed on by fathers and mothers to their unborn fetus. Most pregnant women consume cow's milk, meat, and other acid forming foods. This practice adds to the mother's toxicity and acid load which further increases tissue weakness that is passed on to the unborn fetus.

When our body becomes acidic from the food and drinks we consume, inflammation occurs and nutrients in the blood and the tissues in our body cluster together − a condition called *coagulation*. When the nutrients coagulate or cluster together, our cells cannot use them. They can become *free radicals* which can damage our cells. The acidic foods we eat also produce mucus and congestion, which becomes obstructive. Examples of this obstruction are sinus blockages, sore throats, blurred vision, and much more.

Inflammation

Inflammation is a normal response of the body to any threats, insults, trauma, attacks, or infections. Inflammation causes obstructions and blockages too; pain and swelling are physical signs which result. When inflammation occurs, our immune system reacts by sending white blood cells to combat the insult. An example of chronic inflammation is in Autoimmune Diseases such as Rheumatoid Arthritis, Psoriasis, Diabetes type 1, Ankylosing Spondylitis, Thyroiditis, Multiple Sclerosis, Inflammatory Bowel Diseases, and more. When we have Autoimmune Disorders, our immune system does not distinguish between healthy tissues and potentially harmful antigens. Subsequently, the body sets off a reaction that destroys normal tissues which appears to have similar arrangement as the original threat causing harmful damage, chronic inflammation and pain to our body.

Detoxification is an answer to improving and minimizing inflammation. Alkalization is the method by which detoxification starts. Detoxification not only alkalizes our body, but also gives our body the added energy it needs to clean and heal itself. Fresh fruits and vegetables when eaten are alkalizing to the body. A plant-based diet is low in cholesterol and saturated fats, however, it is high in fiber and antioxidants which is healthy for our body and decreases our risk of chronic diseases.

Gut Health

Poor gut health is the root of many diseases and health problems. The gastrointestinal tract is where digestion, absorption, and elimination takes place. Any negative change to how the gastrointestinal tract functions can be detrimental to life. The process of getting energy from foods begins in our mouth. The colon is where we eliminate our wastes, which is vital to the survival of our body. Proper elimination of wastes, from food digestion and cellular metabolism, is just as important as the ingestion of our foods.

Our bowels take the most abuse from acid-toxic foods and drinks. These foods inflame and weaken the bowel structure. Some foods (like refined starch, refined sugar, and dairy) act like glue and adhere to the walls of the gastrointestinal tract. Other foods (like animal protein) are abrasive and in order to protect itself from further injury, the intestinal walls will produce excessive mucus. This excess mucus will affect the gastrointestinal tract lining and cause disruption in how it processes the digestion and absorption of food.

The gastrointestinal tract also plays a valuable role with the lymphatic system. The lymphatic system is our body's self-cleaning system. The kidneys, the gastrointestinal tract, and the skin are the main outlets the lymphatic system uses to get rid of wastes and toxins from our body. When the skin, kidneys, and colon become impacted or obstructed, the lymphatic system becomes backed up and disease symptoms can occur. We can decongest our body and lymphatic system by detoxifying our temple (body) by using fresh fruits and vegetables to obtain a healthy equilibrium.

Focus Point

Are you experiencing inflammation or gut health problems?

If so, write your symptoms down.

Chapter Four

Understanding the Process of Digestion to Elimination

Digestion

D igestion begins in the mouth with the teeth breaking down the food into smaller pieces. Enzymes, from the salivary glands in the mouth (amylase), are secreted to further break down food into a bolus. A bolus is the mixture of chewed food and saliva within your mouth. After you swallow the bolus, it travels down the esophagus and into the stomach. In the stomach, the initial digestion of protein starts via an enzyme called pepsin. Pepsin is released by hydrochloric acid in the stomach; therefore, pepsin is an acidic enzyme and the stomach is an acidic environment.

After the initial digestion of protein in the stomach, the food bolus, or chyme, travels to the first part of the small intestine, or duodenum, where the majority of digestion continues to take place. In the duodenal section of the small intestine, the pancreas releases sodium bicarbonate, which neutralizes the acid bolus that came from the stomach. The pancreas also secretes digestive enzymes which further helps break down carbohydrates, fats, and proteins. The liver and gallbladder are located in the abdominal cavity on the upper right side. The liver produces bile, a green substance, which is stored in the gallbladder. Bile is released in the digestion process into the duodenum to help emulsify (break down) fats. The small intestine also releases some digestive

31

enzymes that continue the process of breaking down the food into simple components.

After the food is digested, the nutrients from the food are absorbed from the small intestine into the blood. Carbohydrates break down into *simple sugars* that the body uses for fuel. Proteins break down to *simple amino acids* that the body uses for building and repairing. Fats break down into *fatty acids* and *glycerol* for building, repairing, and emergency needs.

In the process of digestion, the mouth is alkaline, the stomach is acidic, and the small intestine is alkaline in nature. When the foods we eat are not properly broken down, we experience gas formation from fermentation and/or decay. Some of the reasons the foods we eat may not be broken down properly can be because of a weak pancreas (weak or deficient enzymes and hormone release), a weak stomach (weak hydrochloric acid), a weak liver or gallbladder (removed gallbladder, gallstones, fatty liver, or diseased liver), a weak intestinal tract, and/or improper food combinations. Digestion is the first step in the food breakdown process that must take place in a healthy body. When we are not digesting properly, because of some of the reasons listed above, this can cause many of us to be vitamin and mineral deficient.

Absorption

When foods are digested and broken down into their respective simple components, the nutrients must be absorbed from the small pores all along the mucous membranes of the small and large intestines into the bloodstream. From the bloodstream, the nutrients can be actively transported or passively diffused in the cells via a wall surrounding the cell called the *cell membrane*. The nutrients which enter the cells go through further processing to be utilized or stored as cell energy. Cell energy is known as Adenosine Triphosphate (ATP). ATP energy is used by the body for fuel, building, repairing, and/or storage for emergency use.

Absorption should be simple. However, problems occur when many years of eating wrong food combinations takes a toll on our body. Our intestines become congested and obstructed with by-products. These by-products come from refined sugars, meats, dairy products, and refined carbohydrates. The by-products cause congestion and impaction from *excessive mucus production* that accumulate within the walls of the intestines. When this mucus congestion and impaction occurs, it eventually blocks or decreases the absorption of the nutritional components from the foods we eat. Subsequently, nutritional, vitamin, and mineral deficiencies result from insufficiencies in the absorption process which eventually leads to leaky gut. A leaky and/or unhealthy gut can be the gateway for many diseases we develop.

Utilization

The bloodstream is the transport system that carries nutrition *to* our cells and *through* our cells. Most of the absorbed nutrients initially goes to the liver for further processing before it goes to the rest of the body for utilization. The liver carries out a number of processes such as creating its own amino acids, changing sugars to fats and fats to sugars, and creating cholesterol from scratch. The liver is an amazing organ that has the ability to build or reconstruct compounds.

Most of the foods commonly eaten by humans are acid forming. When our body becomes acidic from the foods that we eat, the nutrients (such as amino acids, fats, sugars, minerals, and other components) stick or clump together. Cell membrane walls have tiny holes for nutrients to be absorbed through them into the cells. Therefore, these 'clumped' nutrients which are larger than the size of the small cell membrane openings makes absorption of these "clumped nutrients" through the membrane wall difficult. When red blood cells start clumping together, it blocks proper oxygen transport and utilization to the cells. Ultimately, the cells starve which causes glands and organs to function below their limit. It also causes loss of systemic energy, loss of muscle tissue, and finally death of the cell.

Acidity also causes inflammation in the walls of the blood vessels and throughout the body. Once inflammation occurs, our body prompts the liver to make cholesterol (which is anti-inflammatory). Cholesterol is the most common anti-inflammatory lipid that the body uses to fight inflammation. Over time, when the tissues become acidic and inflamed, the liver will produce more cholesterol to fight the inflammation. The cholesterol or lipids (fats) begin sticking to the walls of the blood vessels in an attempt to buffer the inflammation. Ultimately, the continual process of cholesterol buffering the inflammation in the blood vessels and sticking together will decrease the lumen of the blood vessels. Once the lumen of the blood vessel is decreased, blood pumps harder to get through the space, which ultimately results in elevated blood pressure and eventually heart disease. During this time, blood cholesterol levels can also become elevated.

Throughout the body when the lipid binds and clogs together, it can form lipid stones, which can eventually lead to liver and gallbladder stones. In addition to lipids sticking together, minerals can also bind and clump together to form rock-like stones which can lead to kidney stones, gout and/or bone spurs.

Many glands and organs in the body supply hormones and steroids to assist the cells in using different nutrients and minerals for cellular activities. As the glands become hypo-active or underactive from the acid forming foods we consume, the utilization of minerals by cells are affected which creates many disease symptoms. For example, one of the jobs of calcium is to help transport nutrients across the cell membrane walls. The thyroid and/or parathyroid glands regulate calcium levels in the body. When these glands are not functioning efficiently, it can slow or stop calcium utilization by the cells. This dysregulation can cause a domino effect causing the cells to starve. When the cells starve, the tissue can become weak, and the cycle continues until the cells eventually die. Therefore, proper nutrition and food combination is important and translates into how our body and cells utilize nutrients and minerals efficiently for overall health.

Elimination

A healthy gut leads to vitality of the body. Our body has to be efficient in elimination. Our body can eliminate through the colon (stool), the kidneys (urine) and the skin (fever, sweat, and/or rash). Our body is always trying to eliminate in ways that we often do not understand. Examples of elimination could be rash on the body, cold and flu-like symptoms (such as sneezing, coughing and wheezing), sweating, body aches, fevers, and diarrhea. The body uses elimination processes to purge itself of mucus, parasites, toxins, and much more.

We should not see undigested foods in our stools. When we eat food, after our body digests and absorbs the nutrients, by-products of the foods we eat are eliminated via the colon. Our cells after utilizing the nutrients must also excrete by-products. This waste is excreted into the fluids around the cells (called interstitial fluid). By-products such as gasses, acids, cellular wastes, undigested proteins, and unused material (such as vitamins and minerals) must leave our body.

Many of us suffer from constipation. Constipation can be harsh on our body. If we are unable to eliminate wastes, toxins and other by-products of digestion, it can cause congestion of the cells which can lead to cell decay and death. The effects of constipation can also trigger the bowels to release toxins and unwanted by-products back into the bloodstream. The reabsorption of toxins into the blood can cause harmful effects and lead to such diseases as leaky gut, autoimmune disorders, gout, and increased risk of colon cancer and more.

Increased bowel movements (four to six times or more a day) can be concerning as well. This can be a sign of Irritable Bowel Syndrome (IBS). IBS means inflammation of the bowels which can be just as harmful as constipation. When inflammation of IBS occurs, we may not absorb nutrients efficiently from our digested foods. This can lead to malabsorption and ultimately result in cell starvation and death.

The foods we eat, specifically animal flesh products, dairy products (milk and cheese), and refined sugar (found in drinks, cakes, pastries, cookies, ice cream) produce acidosis in our bodies (they are acid forming foods). The acidosis causes inflammation resulting in physical symptoms such as pain and swelling. These acid forming foods cause congestion, obstruction, coagulation of nutrients, free radicals, formation of liver and gallbladder stones, formation of kidney stones, gout, and bone spurs from coagulation of minerals. The inflammation can also cause elevated cholesterol, cholesterol plaque in the blood vessel walls, elevated blood pressure, risk of heart disease, and heart attack. Other chronic diseases associated with the acid forming foods we eat are cancers, autoimmune disease, Polycystic Ovarian Syndrome (PCOS), endometriosis, other female reproductive disorders, decreased libido, erectile dysfunction, and other male reproductive disorders.

In conclusion, to correct and improve these associated medical conditions, we need to dramatically decrease or eliminate entirely these acid forming foods from our diet. It is important to clean, strengthen, and regenerate our cells and tissues. We can do this by detoxifying and regenerating our body and cells with fresh fruits and vegetables.

Detoxification is a process we must go through. Detoxification, naturally, begins as we alkalize our body through a raw food diet with fruits and vegetables. This process strengthens cells by removing the obstructions and acids that cause inflammation and block nutrition to our cells. Detoxification allows cells to gain nutritional energy and to properly eliminate wastes via cellular respiration. Then this begins the rebuilding (regeneration) process within our body.

Adequate or effective elimination means moving your bowels one to three times a day, urinating adequately, sweating, and breathing properly. All of us fail in this category to some extent. By correcting the problems associated with digestion, absorption, utilization, and elimination, we can regain energy, build vitality and wellness while living a disease-free life.

Focus Point

Write down the disease conditions that you are struggling with?

Don't be discouraged, know that by the end of this book, you will learn how to heal your body with the right food choices and combinations.

Chapter Five

Carbohydrates and Diabetes Mellitus

Are Carbohydrates bad for you?

There is a misconception that carbohydrates are bad for us. Most of us are under the assumption that we cannot eat carbohydrates because they make us gain weight. Carbohydrates are not bad for us, however, it is important to note that all carbohydrates are not created equal. Carbohydrates (starch) breaks down to fructose, glucose, and galactose which is utilized by the body as fuel.

Carbohydrates fall into two categories, simple and complex carbohydrates. Simple carbohydrates can be healthy and/or unhealthy. Complex carbohydrates can also be healthy and/or unhealthy. Healthy simple and complex carbohydrates are not refined or processed. Unhealthy simple and complex carbohydrates are most often processed and refined, lacking in adequate nutrients, vitamins, and minerals for our body when consumed.

Examples of healthy simple carbohydrates

All raw and cooked Fruits and Vegetables.

Examples of unhealthy Simple carbohydrates

Table sugar, candy, soda, juice from concentrate, etc.

Examples of *healthy complex* carbohydrates

Rice, Potatoes, Quinoa, Beans, Legumes, etc.

Examples of *unhealthy complex* carbohydrates

Pasta, cakes, cookies, ice cream, potato chips, cereal, etc.

Simple carbohydrates that are healthy, such as fresh fruits and vegetables, are not processed. They are also composed of fiber which helps slow down digestion and the rate at which insulin is released. Once digested, they provide the body with important nutrients, vitamins, minerals, antioxidants, and more. These healthy simple carbohydrates also promote a healthy gut and lead to regularity of the bowels instead of causing constipation.

Simple carbohydrates that are unhealthy, such as table sugar are processed. These carbohydrates do not have fiber. Once ingested and digested, they can raise the blood sugar and insulin level fast because there is no fiber to slow down the digestion process with its effect on the cells and body. They have no nutritional value and cause acidosis and inflammation in the body which can lead to insulin resistance and many other chronic diseases.

Therefore, the answer to the question, "Are carbohydrates bad for you?" is "Yes" and "No". If we want to obtain health, vitality and wellness, it is crucial that we eat more of the *healthy, unprocessed simple and complex* carbohydrates. When we choose to eat unhealthy, processed, simple and complex carbohydrates we increase our risk of developing chronic diseases and premature death over time.

It is important to eat fruits and vegetables (simple carbohydrates) in its natural form instead of cooking it. If it must be cooked, then it should be cooked and eaten with no added fats. For example, they can be (boiled, stir-fried, baked, broiled or air fried).

Understanding Food Combinations

Understanding food combinations is very important. For example, starchy carbohydrates should be eaten with vegetables which have fiber to help with digestion and minimize an increased glycemic response. Starchy carbohydrates should not be eaten with animal products. Although we discourage the consumption of animal products, if you must eat it, combine them with vegetables instead of starchy carbohydrates. Improper food combinations can affect our digestion and elimination process. Not combining food properly can cause many unwanted symptoms such as gas, bloating, acid reflux, headaches, inflammation (pain and swelling) and more.

Can Diabetics Eat Fruits?

This is another question we hear a lot. To understand this question we have to understand how the body processes the food that we eat. We have to understand how the body develops Diabetes Mellitus and the different types of Diabetes Mellitus.

What are the different type of Diabetes mellitus?

Diabetes mellitus is when the blood sugar is consistently high in our blood stream for a long period of time and causes metabolic problems. There is a correlation between elevated blood sugar and insulin. When the body senses an elevation of glucose in the blood, the body signals the pancreas gland to secrete insulin from its beta cells. Insulin secreted into the bloodstream travels to the targeted cells to help in getting glucose into the cells for the cells to utilize it and produce ATP. Insulin does this by binding to receptors on the cell membrane (it is like a lock and key) to open the gate for the glucose to be transported across the cell membrane into the cell.

Over years of eating poorly, such as eating a diet full of saturated fat, processed food, refined carbohydrates and high protein, our body gets acidotic and inflamed. Our pancreas, adrenal glands and other organs and glands get fatigued from working so hard to sustain our poor eating habits.

We also develop an accumulation of fat in our cells (specifically our liver and muscle cells). This accumulation of fat in the cells causes the cells to send a signal to the receptors on the cell membrane to stop accepting food energy into the cells because it has enough energy. When this occurs, the receptor resists insulin and does not allow insulin to bind to it even though there is a high level of sugar (glucose) in the blood waiting to get into the cell. Therefore, the receptor is resistant to the insulin, causing *insulin resistance*. As the body continues to remain insulin resistant, Pre-Diabetes, Diabetes Mellitus type 2 and other chronic diseases develop.

We can improve our health and become *insulin sensitive*. The body and the cells can utilize the carbohydrates that we consume efficiently and improve our DM II or even reverse it. We need to become efficient at utilizing the fat that has accumulated in our cells. One way to do this is by *water fasting*. When we fast from food, our blood sugar levels and insulin levels go down. The body will utilize the fat we have accumulated and thus start making us insulin sensitive over time.

Another way is to eat a *low fat diet*. Unprocessed fruits and vegetables have lots of fiber, nutrients, vitamins and minerals. They are also low in fat and when eaten the body utilizes its nutrients and burns the accumulated stored fat in the cells thus improving insulin resistance. Specifically fruits are high in antioxidants and they break down relatively fast to *fructose*. Fruits require very little energy to metabolize. Fructose moves into the cell passively for the nutrients, vitamins and minerals to be utilized, requiring very little energy to get inside the cells. Fructose can be transported into the cells without the help of insulin making it a healthy food for diabetics to consume and improve insulin resistance.

There are several types of diabetes but there are two main types that we will discuss in this book: DM type I and DM type II.

Diabetes Mellitus type I (Insulin Dependent) is most often an autoimmune problem and requires insulin for management. Diabetes Mellitus Type II is a metabolic problem that most of the time does not require insulin.

Diabetes mellitus Type I

This type of Diabetes affects about 10% of people in the world. This is an *autoimmune disease* where a large percentage of the beta-cells of the pancreas have been destroyed through genetic factors, environmental factors, and immunological factors. The problem is that the pancreas is not able to secrete insulin because of the auto destruction of the beta cells of the pancreas. Therefore for this type of Diabetes, exogenous insulin (insulin from outside the body) is needed. There are genetic, environmental, and immunologic factors that can contribute to the development of autoimmune diseases.

Genetic Factors

We inherit both strong and weakened genes from our parents. There are genetic factors such as genetically susceptible genes that predispose people to the autoimmune destruction of the Beta cells of the pancreas causing Diabetes Mellitus Type I. The autoimmune destruction process can occur over a period of months to years during which we have no symptoms or blood sugar problems until a significant amount of the beta cells in the pancreas are destroyed for us to become symptomatic. Therefore, in DM type I, the problem is that the pancreas cannot release insulin because there has been a destruction of the beta cells.

Environmental Factors

Environmental factors that can cause auto-antibody destruction of the beta cells of the pancreas can be infections (such as viruses), toxins, and nutrients (such as foreign proteins) from the acidic foods that we eat.

Immunological Factors

Immunological factors can be when the body mounts an immune response towards a foreign body such as viruses and foreign protein (found in animal protein, cheese, cow's milk, and gluten, etc) which comes into the body from the foods we eat. The antibodies created are not specific and can also be directed against antigens that have similar molecular sequences located on various organs and glands in the body (for example: thyroid, pancreas, joints, muscles, etc). This is mainly how autoimmune diseases (which can be highly inflammatory and debilitating) develop.

Diabetes mellitus Type II

This type of Diabetes is the most common type affecting many people worldwide. It is a metabolic problem coming from our poor dietary intake. The problem is not the pancreas ability to secrete insulin. Insulin is released normally by the pancreas in response to elevation of blood sugar. The problem is that the receptors on the cell membrane resist the insulin because of a number of things, but specifically it is due to having too much dietary fat accumulation in the cells.

In both types of diabetes, proper diet and exercise can help them improve health, vitality and wellness.

When a Type I diabetic eats a diet high in fruits, vegetables and other wholesome plant based foods, they improve their insulin resistance and become insulin sensitive. As they become insulin sensitive, their insulin requirement decreases and they use less insulin and overtime their A1c improves. However, Type I Diabetics, even a healthy diet, will still require lifelong treatment with insulin.

Type II Diabetics as they become insulin sensitive with whole plant foods, will notice a decrease in their daily blood sugar monitoring relatively quickly. Their A1c over time will also improve. Overtime with proper diet and exercise under the direction and supervision of their Provider, most type II Diabetics can improve and/or reverse their diabetes diagnosis requiring little or no medications.

Both Type I and Type II Diabetics, as they improve with proper diet and nutrition, will decrease their risk of other chronic diseases such as kidney problems, eye problems, heart disease, neuropathy and much more including premature death.

Most diets or eating plans agree that processed simple carbohydrates such as white sugar, soft drinks, and other refined carbohydrates such as breads, cakes, cookies, and pies are not good for us. These foods lack fiber and nutrients which cause a rapid spike or rise in our blood sugar because there is no fiber to buffer it. These simple carbohydrates, unlike fruits, make us feel hungry sooner. The short-lived fullness leads to overeating, weight gain, and conditions like diabetes mellitus type II, high blood pressure, and so forth. Therefore, we want to consume whole foods (such as simple and complex carbohydrates found in fruits, vegetables, whole grains, potatoes, beans and legumes) in their most natural state. These foods are digested and processed slowly in our body. They have lots of other nutrients such as vitamins, minerals, phytonutrients, and fiber which helps with digestion and elimination. When we eat a low-fat whole food plant-based diet, we decrease the fat content and increase the fiber content in our diet. A healthy diet with raw fruits and vegetables will alkalize and detoxify our body allowing regeneration of our cells to take place which will improve our overall wellbeing and vitality.

Our body is constantly working, and it needs energy to use to maintain the function of our body. Our body uses carbohydrates as the primary source of energy for the brain, nervous system, blood cells, and muscles. Therefore, if we do not eat fat, our body is going to break down the fat we have stored in our body and use it to maintain our body's function. If we eat a lot of fat in our diet, the body is going to utilize the fat from the diet first instead of the fat that is stored in our body. The incoming fat goes into the cells without the aid of insulin, and the fat clogs up the function of our cell system creating free radicals which causes inflammation throughout our body.

Another function of insulin is to store fat into the fat cells and muscle cells; therefore, the greater amount of insulin that is in the bloodstream, the more fat we will store.

How do we decrease glucose and insulin levels in the blood?

Fasting

Fasting gets the insulin and glucose levels down in the blood. Water fasting is the absence of food and the ingestion of water for a short period of time. We can fast for a few hours or a few days. Prolonged water fasting, 24 hours or longer should be medically supervised.

Fasting for shorter periods of time during the day is what is known as intermittent fasting. When we sleep, our body goes into fasting mode, the insulin level decreases in the bloodstream, and our body uses this time to repair and heal itself. Therefore, the first meal we consume after waking up is considered breaking the fast. To prolong the fast, extend the time we wait to eat our first meal. This will allow our body to continue to heal and repair itself. For example, if we stopped eating our last meal at 6 in the evening and consumed our first meal at 8 in the morning, we would have fasted for 14 hours. If we want to increase the fasting hours, then we can push eating our first meal until 10 in the morning. This will give us 16 hours of fasting. Then we eat our meals between 10 in the morning to 6 in the evening which is a period of 8 hours. This routine is what is known as 16:8 intermittent fasting. This type of fasting is safe for most people, however, approach it with caution and under the supervision of your doctor.

During periods of fasting, glycogen (stored glucose molecules within cells) is used as fuel when glucose and insulin level decreases. The body will break down stored glycogen (from liver and muscle cells) into glucose and release it into the bloodstream to be utilized as fuel in a process known as *glycogenolysis*. Likewise, the body can produce new glucose from non-carbohydrate precursors to be used as fuel in a process known as *gluconeogenesis*. The body also uses stored fats in the cells to be used for energy. This promotes weight loss. Weight loss decreases the secretion of the molecule adipokine which attaches to glycoprotein receptors on cell membranes. The decrease in the effect of the molecule adipokine reduces inflammation and improves insulin resistance.

Low Fat Diet

A low-fat high carbohydrate whole food plant-based diet (which is a diet high in whole fruits, vegetables, grains, legumes, nuts and seeds - consumed in its most natural state) works best because when we decrease the fat in our diet daily, this allows the cells in the body, specifically the liver and skeletal muscles, to use the fat that has accumulated inside the cells. The utilization of excessive fat inside the cells makes the glycoprotein receptors (on the surface of the cells) become more sensitive to the binding of insulin, thus the term insulin sensitivity. Insulin sensitivity promotes weight loss and decreases the release of the cytokines by the adipose tissue (which causes damage to our body).

High Protein Diet

A high protein diet eliminates refined carbohydrates (which is good) but increases the consumption of large amounts of animal protein and fats which puts stress on the kidneys. A high protein diet is low in fiber, which causes constipation, allowing free radicals to roam throughout our body which cause cell damage, illness, and premature aging and inflammation of our body. Eating a high protein diet can help us lose weight and may improve our diabetic numbers but it does not lower our risk of heart attack, inflammation, high cholesterol, stone formation, nor cellular starvation.

Exercise

A healthy diet with regular exercise is especially important to help improve insulin resistance and decrease our weight and/or keep our weight in control by burning fat from muscle cells. Exercise increases our muscle mass which burns more calories while we sleep. Exercise increases endorphins and makes us feel and sleep better.

Hydration

Our body is at least 70% water. Our body is designed to utilize water to help replenish us and use water to cleanse our body of toxins and wastes. Without adequate hydration like plain water we increase the risk of dehydration. This also causes toxins to be reabsorbed which can lead to serious complications and problems in our body. Therefore, it is important to get adequate hydration into the body for optimum wellness. There are some people who are under water restriction by their physicians because of their medical conditions (such as patients with congestive heart failure). These people need to follow the advice of their doctor as to how much water they can drink.

Rest

Our body needs rest and relaxation to reboot and re-energize. It is important to get adequate and restful sleep and to take time to rest and relax to enjoy things that bring peace and equilibrium to our mind and body.

Sunlight

Getting necessary sunlight is crucial for certain processes and functions in our body. When we do not get adequate sunlight, our body can become deficient in certain vitamins that help to heal and protect our body.

Therefore, it is important to note that in addition to food, getting enough rest and relaxation, exercise, adequate hydration, sunlight and a healthy mindset all contributes to cultivating a healthy spirit, soul and body.

Focus Point

Are you a Diabetic?

Have you been told you cannot eat fruits?

Are you convinced that fruits are healthy for you and you can start incorporating fruits into your diet regimen?

51

Chapter Six

Insulin Resistance

Insulin is a hormone that is secreted by the Beta cells of the pancreas (which is one of the organs in our body). Insulin helps control the amount of sugar (glucose) in the blood. Insulin regulates the metabolism of carbohydrates by promoting the absorption of glucose (sugar) from the blood into cells. Glucose gives us energy, however, too much glucose can be harmful to our health. The foods we eat are composed of macronutrients such as carbohydrates, proteins, and/or fats. In this chapter of Insulin Resistance, we will focus on carbohydrate metabolism.

Carbohydrate Metabolism

Carbohydrate metabolism starts in the mouth. The saliva has an enzyme in it that starts the breakdown of carbohydrate (which is starch). The broken-down starch is transferred to the stomach and then to the small intestines (our gut) for further digestion. In the small intestines more enzymes are released by the pancreas to further break down the carbohydrate (starch) to glucose. The glucose is absorbed into the blood from the pores along the small intestines.

When glucose is absorbed into the blood from the small intestine, there is a high level of glucose in the bloodstream after a carbohydrate rich meal. In a healthy body, our body signals the pancreas to release insulin into the blood to help move the high glucose in the blood from the blood into the cells. Our body's preferred source of energy is glucose; therefore, our body wants to get the glucose from the blood into the cells where it can be used for energy.

What causes Insulin Resistance?

Insulin Resistance is sometimes referred to as impaired glucose tolerance or metabolic syndrome. Metabolic Syndrome includes a group of problems associated with *obesity, high blood pressure, high cholesterol,* and *type 2 diabetes.* There are many factors that cause insulin resistance, however, one of the common factors of insulin resistance is too much *"fat"* in our diet. When we have insulin resistance, our pancreas makes more insulin to make up for the elevated "sugar" in our blood. For a while this works and our body blood sugar levels remain normal. Over time, our pancreas will not be able to keep up with the demand if we do not make changes in the way we eat and exercise. If our poor eating habits stay the same, our blood sugar levels will rise until we develop pre-diabetes and eventually diabetes. The end result of insulin resistance is *"elevated blood sugar"* and *"elevated insulin in the blood"*. However, the root cause of insulin resistance is the high dietary fat that we consistently eat. Excessive intracellular fat (which means our cells are full of fat), slows down glucose uptake into our cells by causing the receptors to resist the binding of insulin to it. Therefore, a high dietary fat causes an excess of glucose and insulin to become elevated in the bloodstream.

On the surface of "cells" are receptors called glycoprotein receptors. The hormone "insulin" binds to these glycoprotein receptors so that glucose in the blood can be actively transported into the cells to be utilized for energy (this is a normal process). Food energy and cell energy are different. Food energy comes from the food we eat. Carbohydrates break down to sugar, proteins break down to amino acids and fats break down to fatty acids and glycerol, these are examples of food energy. Food energy transports inside the cell to be utilized in producing "cell energy" known as Adenosine Triphosphate (ATP) through a series of complicated processes that the body can use.

What happens when the Glycoprotein Receptors on the cells and the Insulin Process becomes Abnormal?

When the process of insulin binding to the glycoprotein receptors becomes abnormal, "insulin resistance" occurs. When insulin resistance occurs, the problem causes *glucose* and *insulin* to back up and increase in the blood. This results in glucose being inefficiently transported inside our cells. The prolonged buildup of *glucose* and *insulin* in the bloodstream eventually leads to pre-diabetes, and Diabetes mellitus type II.

How Does Obesity Cause Insulin Resistance?

When we are overweight (obese), the overabundance of *fat cells* in our body produces and secretes a *cytokine molecule* known as *adipokine*. Adipokine travels throughout the bloodstream and attaches itself to the glycoprotein receptors on the cell surfaces where insulin is supposed to attach; therefore, it blocks insulin from doing its function of helping to move glucose into the cells. The inability of insulin attaching to the receptors creates a buildup of glucose in the bloodstream.

Another reason the glycoprotein receptors on the cell surface can become inefficient is when we eat too many dietary fats (such as cooking oils, animal protein, dairy such as milk and cheese, fried foods, processed foods, etc.). The dietary fat (just like adipokine) can attach to the glycoprotein receptor and block insulin from attaching to it. Therefore, this leaves a buildup of glucose and insulin in the bloodstream over time eventually causing our body to become pre-diabetic. When poor dietary habits are not corrected, pre-diabetes advances to diabetes.

Most people don't realize they have insulin resistance until they have a blood test done. At times our high blood sugar levels will fluctuate. When our body's sugar level is consistently high, we may notice an increase in thirst, increased urination, fatigue, blurred vision, and/or tingling on the bottom of our feet. Diabetes is a serious condition and can significantly damage the heart, blood vessels, kidneys, eyes and more over time. Some signs of insulin resistance include:

- A fasting glucose level over 100 mg/dL

- Blood pressure readings of 130/80 or higher

- A waistline over 40 inches in men and 35 inches in women

- A fasting triglyceride level over 150 mg/dL

- An HDL cholesterol level under 40 mg/dL in men and 50 mg/dL in women

- Skin Tags

- Patches of dark, velvety skin called acanthosis nigricans

Obesity (being significantly overweight with a high body fat index), an inactive lifestyle, and a diet high in refined carbohydrates and dietary fat are the primary causes of insulin resistance. Certain diseases such as heart disease, nonalcoholic fatty liver disease, hypertension, high cholesterol, and polycystic ovary syndrome are associated with insulin resistance. If insulin resistance or metabolic syndrome goes untreated, it can lead to:

- Heart attack

- Stroke

- Eye problems

- Kidney problems

- Cancer

- Alzheimer's disease

- Blood sugar imbalances (such as severe high and/or low blood sugar)

Insulin Resistance and Chronic Diseases

Insulin Resistance is a risk factor for many chronic diseases such as heart disease, hypertension, high cholesterol, kidney disease, cancers, female hormone imbalance, male reproductive problems, respiratory problems, thyroid problems, liver disease, osteoarthritis, and much more. Insulin resistance may also occur if our adrenal glands are weak.

How do Adipokine Molecules affect other organs and vessels?

Adipokine, as described previously, circulates, and binds to glycoprotein receptors and increases the risk of Pre-Diabetes and Diabetes. Adipokine molecules, as they circulate through the blood, can damage blood vessels, and increase the risk of heart disease. These molecules also damage joints increasing the risk of osteoarthritis.

How do we decrease insulin and glucose from the blood and improve Insulin Resistance?

We must take steps to reverse insulin resistance and prevent type II diabetes along with the risk of other chronic diseases. We must eat a healthy diet that includes a variety of fresh fruits and vegetables. Eating fruits and vegetables in their raw and natural state as much as possible (whole food plant base) will help our body trim down to a healthier weight. We should exercise at least thirty (30) minutes a day with moderate activity if possible, such as brisk walking and resistance training. If we are not active now, we need to work up to that as our body permits.

The best foods to eat are fruits, vegetables, whole grains, and legumes. We also receive healthy fiber as we eat lots of fresh fruits, vegetables and legumes. Over time our cells will use up the fat deposits already stored inside the cells, and glucose uptake into the cells will become efficient again. This process is called *insulin sensitivity*. Eating fresh fruits and vegetables helps us lose weight and improve our blood pressure and other chronic diseases. Stay away from animal products, dairy products, and oils as much as possible. This will increase mucus production, congestion, inflammation and constipation.

Focus Point

What does Insulin Resistance mean to you?

Are you ready to decrease the "fat" in your diet to reverse insulin resistance, lose weight and get healthy?

Write down the changes you plan to make in your diet to accomplish this?

Chapter Seven

Adrenal Glands and Disease Conditions

The foods that we eat affect our body in a negative or positive way. This *physiological* response takes time. Over many years of eating acid forming foods, such as animal flesh, dairy products, refined sugar, and processed foods, the by-products of these foods cause inflammation, excessive mucus production, congestion, obstruction, and coagulation of nutrients causing free radicals, formation of stones (gallbladder stones, liver stones, kidney stones, bone spurs, etc.), elevated cholesterol, cholesterol plaque, elevated blood pressure, heart attacks, cancer, and more. These acid-forming foods eventually weaken our tissues, organs, glands, and cells causing poor performance and function.

<u>The Adrenal Gland</u>

The adrenal glands are two small triangular shaped glands, located on top of each kidney, and have very important functions. The adrenal gland is divided into two parts: the *adrenal cortex* and the *adrenal medulla*. The adrenal glands produce hormones that help regulate metabolism, immune system, blood pressure, response to stress, and other important functions. The adrenal glands not only produce anti-inflammatory steroids, they also produce sexual reproductive steroids like estrogen, testosterone, and progesterone. These steroids are also produced in the ovaries of females (estrogen and progesterone) and in the testis of males (testosterone).

When the adrenal glands become weak with the acid-forming foods we consistently eat, the production and release of the neurotransmitters and steroids will be weak. The weakness of the adrenal glands can also contribute to hormone imbalance in men and women.

Inflammatory Conditions

The *adrenal cortex* produces and secretes steroids. Some of these steroids fight inflammation (anti-inflammatory) like corticosteroids and progesterone. Other steroids are acid-like steroids, they break things down like estrogen, testosterone, and androsterone.

Some of the foods we eat cause acidosis within the body (like animal flesh and dairy). These foods cause inflammation that expresses itself in the form of pain and swelling. When steroids, which fight inflammation (anti-inflammatory), are not produced adequately because of underactive adrenal glands, (secondary to the foods we eat), inflammation occurs in our body. Without the anti-inflammatory effect of steroids, ongoing inflammation occurs throughout our body. If we do not stop consuming the acid-forming foods, which is the root cause of the problem, inflammation will continue to occur.

Some examples of inflammatory conditions are: Colitis, Diverticulitis, Arthritis, Bursitis, Prostatitis, Gout and much more. When we stop consuming the offending foods, inflammation will improve as our body heals itself. The key to this is to stop consuming the offending foods causing inflammation and to start detoxifying our body with alkaline foods such as raw fruits and vegetables.

Female Reproductive Conditions

Estrogen is an acid-type steroid (it breaks things down). Estrogen is produced in the adrenal glands but it is also produced in the ovaries. There are different types of estrogen and some of these types of estrogen can be produced from the liver and fat cells. At the end of the menstrual cycle, estrogen (the main type estradiol) breaks down the lining of the uterus to cause menstrual flow to occur each month.

Progesterone is an anti-inflammatory steroid hormone that counterbalances the effect of estrogen. Progesterone is produced in the adrenal cortex and in the ovaries. The progesterone produced in the ovaries needs a prohormone to be produced. Therefore, if the adrenal gland is weak (from the acid-forming foods we eat), progesterone and the prohormone production level will be low causing the estrogen to be produced in excess quantities from the ovaries with no counterbalance effect of progesterone leading to a condition called *estrogen dominance.*

When we become estrogen dominant (because there is no counterbalance of progesterone), we can experience many female hormone disorders such as:

- Menstrual irregularities

- Excessive bleeding/Abnormal Uterine Bleeding

- Fibrocystic changes/conditions

- Ovarian Cysts

- Uterine Fibroids

- Endometriosis

- Polycystic Ovarian Syndrome (PCOS)

- Conception problems

- Female cancers such as (Breast Cancer, Uterine Cancer & Ovarian Cancer)

We can improve and minimize these conditions by stopping the offending foods that are causing the problems listed above. We should aim to alkalize our body with raw fruits and vegetables. As we do this, our body will start detoxification which removes excess mucus and/or congestion, obstructions, free radicals, and inflammation from our body. Our body will be energized and will promote cellular respiration and cellular regeneration which will revitalize our body and improve our vitality and well-being.

Male Reproductive Conditions

The adrenal cortex produces testosterone, androsterone, and progesterone. Testosterone is also produced in the testis of males from stimulation of the brain. Testosterone and androsterone are acid-like steroid hormones and they are aggressive in creating cellular changes. These steroids are counterbalanced by the anti-inflammatory steroid effect of progesterone.

When the adrenal glands are weak (from the acid-forming foods we eat), there is an underproduction of the steroid progesterone and the prohormone which is made. Testosterone is also produced in the testes therefore, when there is no counterbalance of the testosterone because of the decrease in progesterone, this aggressive male hormone (testosterone) can lead to prostate overstimulation and inflammation. Problems associated with this include:

- Prostatitis

- Prostate Cancer

- Erection Problems

- Decrease Libido

- Low Energy

- Low Endurance

The simple solution to this is to stop the offending agent (the acid-forming foods), alkalize, detoxify, and regenerate the body with a plant based diet.

Carbohydrate Metabolism

There are many hormones that regulate carbohydrate metabolism. Major hormones are insulin and glucagon released by the pancreas, glucocorticoids and catecholamines released by the adrenal gland.

One of the main hormones that gets dysregulated in weakened adrenal glands is cortisol. Cortisol regulates blood sugar. Continued stress with poor eating habits, environmental toxins, and constant stress on the adrenal glands may lead to adrenal fatigue or dysfunction.

Stress response causes cortisol to be elevated in the body which increases blood glucose (without the intake of food). Therefore stress in itself can cause an elevation in cortisol which will increase glucose and cause insulin resistance. This dysregulation causes insulin to increase and Type II diabetes may result from prolonged stress. Stress may also lead to anxiety attacks, sweating, and heart palpitations. These are some of the reasons why managing stress is very important for our overall health and well-being.

We can strengthen our body and mind, by detoxing our body, with alkaline foods such as fresh fruits and vegetables and managing our stress levels.

The Adrenal Medulla

The middle part of the adrenal glands is the adrenal medulla. The adrenal medulla is where neurotransmitters are produced, released, and communicated to many different parts of our body. The main hormones released in the adrenal medulla are epinephrine (adrenaline) and norepinephrine (noradrenaline) which are responsible for the *flight or fight* response (which is how we deal with acute stress). In acute stress, these hormones help in increasing the heart rate, heart contractions, blood vessel constriction, increasing blood flow to the brain and muscles, relaxing the smooth muscles of the airway, and in glucose metabolism. When the acute stressful event is over with, the hormones epinephrine, norepinephrine and cortisol should go back to normal levels. When stress is not managed properly and becomes chronic, these hormones remain elevated and cause many symptoms and problems we experience. Examples of some of the problems that we may experience under chronic stress are neurological dysfunctions (such as tremors and brain fog), anxiety, sleep disturbances, asthma, heart arrhythmias, and constipation. We have to find ways to manage our stress and relax to obtain a better mental, emotional and physical well-being. For example, practice deep breathing exercises. Take in a deep breath and release your breath slowly, blowing it out until all the breath is released out. Repeat this about five to ten times and you will be relaxed.

Focus Point

Write down some things that are stressing you.

Write down some healthy things you can do to help you destress.

(For example: Praying, Exercise, Reading, Dancing, Listening to music, and whatever best fits you).

Chapter Eight

Psychological component of eating

Addiction

Addiction is defined as a neuropsychological disorder characterized by a persistent and intense urge to engage in certain behaviors. Addiction is a serious problem that can ruin lives. Most of us are addicted to something. Addiction can be physical and/or behavioral. Alcohol addiction, Illicit drugs, and Prescription drugs are considered Physical addiction. Behavioral addiction is when we lose control of our actions in order to engage in behaviors that result in brief happiness. We become dependent on the pleasurable feelings that come as a result of certain behaviors and begin to compulsively act on that behavior. Examples of behavioral addictions are food addiction, sex addition, video game addiction, gambling addiction and much more. However, physical and behavioral addictions go hand in hand. We can be addicted to "behaviors" just as seriously as we can become addicted to "substances" such as alcohol and hard drugs. Although drugs, alcohol and tobacco are commonly recognized as addictions, there are many other types of addictions.

Cravings, compulsions, inability to stop and lifestyle dysfunction all point to the existence of some type of addiction. People with addiction engage in behaviors that become compulsive despite substantial harm and other negative consequences. Negative effects with the development of addiction can include financial issues, relationship issues, family conflict and destructive behavior.

The very things that we are addicted to and are searching for are also destroying us. There is usually a void we are trying to fill with our addictions to make up for what we are missing in life. This void will never be filled with our addictions. Only God has the answer to the void that is in us. Therefore, it is important to find and align yourself with the one who has the answer to your problem because He is the KEY!

Types of Addiction

- Alcoholism
- Drug Addiction (Prescription and Illicit drugs)
- Tobacco Addiction
- Pornography & Sex Addition
- Food Addiction
- Video Game Addiction
- Internet Addiction
- Gambling Addiction
- Shopping Addiction
- Work Addiction
- Exercise Addiction

Most addiction is a treatable, chronic medical disease which involves a complex interaction of the mind, genetics, the environment and our life experiences. Upon withdrawal or abstinence from the chronic addictive behavior, activity, or habit-forming substance, a person can develop symptoms such as anxiety, irritability, tremors and nausea. Most physical and behavioral addictions are treatable by Professionals and with family and community support. Therefore, do not lose hope, get the help you need and deserve.

Psychological component to eating

In this chapter, we will focus on food addiction and ways to combat the psychological component of eating. There is a huge psychological component to eating and it most likely started at a young age. As children our parents and loved ones told us to eat everything on our plate. We probably also had some traumas or negative experiences where food was used as comfort. Therefore, we developed an unhealthy relationship with food, such as eating when we were not hungry and/or eating unhealthy foods for emotional comfort.

The biggest challenge in incorporating fruits and vegetables into a health journey is dealing with previous eating habits of animal proteins, dairy, refined carbohydrates, and saturated fats. These foods taste good to the palate and are convenient to find. However, chicken, beef, or fish by itself does not taste good without seasoning or salt. Breaking old eating habits is hard because many of us are emotional eaters. We live to eat instead of eating to live. Breaking old eating habits may feel like we are grieving. Grieving is good because it is part of the healing process which is necessary for good health and freedom. There is also another challenge which is the social aspect. These foods are addictive. They are being advertised all around us (television commercials, billboards, and on social media). It takes renewing the mind to accept that nature has given us everything we need in terms of nutritious food.

Emotional Eating is real.

Why do we Emotionally Eat?

- Boredom

- Guilt

- Anger

- Frustration

- Worry

- Fear

- Sadness and much more.

What steps can we take to get a better handle on Emotional Eating?

1. First of all, we have to be aware and accept the fact that we are emotional eaters in order to do something about it. We all get emotional about something.

2. Before we put food, alcohol, cigarettes, or drugs in our mouth, ask," am I eating because I am hungry or am I abusing my body because I am emotionally stressed, frustrated, or angry about something or with someone?" Checking our emotional status is important, because if

it is not true hunger, our emotional state is going to lead us into the "I don't care mode," where we eat whatever we want (comfort junk food full of refined sugar, refined carbohydrates, processed food, fats, and salt). After we consume the food, later we feel a sense of guilt and our body may become bloated, retain fluid, constipated, sinus issues, headaches, and more. The emotional circumstance that caused the unhealthy eating, heavy alcohol consumption, excessive smoking, and/or illegal drug use will still be there. Now these psychological problems can advance to become physical problems.

3. The emotional component of health and stress can take a toll on our blood pressure, heart, mindset, gut, and general well-being. Stress and emotions can also play havoc on our internal hormones like cortisol, insulin, estrogen, and a whole host of hormones that become imbalanced which triggers negative effects in our body. Next time when we get emotional, frustrated, worried, upset or fearful about something, let's take a deep breath, go for a walk, clear our minds, and get better control over our emotions before we start eating for comfort or doing something unhealthy.

4. We need to write things down in a journal. We need to write about the things that caused the sad, frustrated, worried, bored, scared, and angry emotions and what was done to improve our feelings. Stress and emotional things occur every day, but our response to the stress or emotional triggers, is the key to our success and victory. In our journal, let's face the emotions head on. Writing the feelings down exposes the emotion. Speak boldly to

the emotion and tell that emotion to take a back seat. In doing so, the emotion cannot wreak havoc in our lives. We have to expose the emotion in order to dispose of it. We have more control and power than we give ourselves credit. After the emotion has been identified, let's focus on positive thoughts and choose positivity.

5. Memorize one scripture that you can repeat during the day. For example: "I can do all things through Christ which strengthens me." (Philippians 4:13).

6. Reward the overcoming of the emotion. Put a dollar in a bowl every time an unwanted emotion is overcome. By the end of the week, we may have at least 10 dollars to reward ourselves in a healthy way.

7. In dealing with snacking, pick a sweet fruit (such as frozen grapes) to eat or a vegetable (such as crunchy carrots) if needed to munch on. By doing this, it will be hard to overeat by consuming such healthy foods.

8. Practice deep breathing exercises. Take in a deep breath and release your breath slowly, blowing it out until all the breath is released out. Repeat this about five to ten times and you will be relaxed. This will help you think clearly and make wise decisions.

9. Get Professional counseling if needed because an unstable emotional well-being affects mental and physical well-being.

10. What we face during a particular time determines the importance of what we value most. For example, if we

do not have money, what we value most in life will be trying to acquire money. On the other hand, if we have money but have poor health then we would probably value obtaining better health. Money is good and can help us obtain the luxuries of life but it cannot buy our life back when we are dying. Therefore, obtaining good health, vitality and wellness is priceless.

Positive Affirmations

Words have power. Positive affirmations with words can shift our thought patterns, bringing in power, confidence, positive energy, love, compassion and a positive boost to our mental health and well-being. The Bible says, *"So then faith cometh by hearing, and hearing by the word of God."* (Romans 10:17). We are made in the image of God, therefore all good things the Bible says about us is true. With positive word affirmation, we develop faith and thus believe.

Do not let anyone, past or present experiences affect us negatively because we are of value to God. Reject people's negative words to you as well as your own negative words to yourself. Let us *shift our mindset* and *choose positivity*. Please take some time every day to speak positive word affirmations to yourself. When we speak these words enough times, we will start to believe them.

Example of Positive affirmations:

- I am beautiful or handsome.
- I love me.
- I choose me.

- I am more than enough.
- I am of value.
- I am smart.
- I am happy.
- I choose joy.
- I choose peace.
- I am wealthy.
- I deserve it.
- I am worth it.
- I can do and will do it.
- I look and feel radiant.
- I choose health.
- I love fruits.
- I love vegetables.
- I choose God and I choose me.

Speak anything else positive that comes to you.

Focus Point

Write down some of your emotional triggers which cause you to eat unhealthy foods?

Write down some things you can do to counteract your triggers.

Practice deep breathing exercises. Take in a deep breath and release your breath slowly, blowing it out until all the breath is released out. Repeat this about five to ten times and you will be relaxed.

Chapter Nine

The Renew Health Transformation Program (RHTP)

What? know ye not that your body is the temple of the Holy Ghost which is in you, which ye have of God, and ye are not your own? For ye are bought with a price: therefore glorify God in your body, and in your spirit, which are God's.

(1 Corinthians 6: 19-20)

What is the Renew Health Transformation Program?

The Renew Health Transformation Program focuses on using plant based whole food nutrition and natural herbs for the healing of the body to increase vitality and wellness. The Renew Health Transformation Program helps you lose weight in a healthy and sustainable manner, minimize or eliminate medications, improve quality sleep, decrease inflammation and pain, improve mental clarity and cognition, improve gut health, therefore increasing vitality and well-being. Everything in life worth having takes discipline, commitment and consistency. By approaching the Renew Health Transformation Program with such principles and dedication, success will be obtained. On this program, we teach you about proper food combinations.

The Renew Health Transformation Program is structured into *fruit days* and **vegetable days**. If health, healing and weight loss is your goal, we recommend you follow *option one*. If health and healing is your goal but you do not want to lose weight then follow *option two*.

The emphasis of this lifestyle journey is to promote and incorporate low-fat whole food plant-based meals into our diet. Many diets and fitness journeys can help us lose weight however, what this program is about is not just about weight loss but about promoting a healthy lifestyle and preventing and healing our bodies of chronic diseases. Ultimately, we have to choose a healthy journey that fits our lifestyle and health needs.

There are many opinions on one diet versus another. One thing all mainstream diets agree on is the fact that refined carbohydrates and processed foods (such as cakes, cookies, soft drinks, candy, chips and ice cream) are not healthy to eat. This book is not written to be critical of other diet plans but to bring forth a healthy lifestyle that is natural, easy, effortless and sustainable in achieving optimum health.

Initially, this eating regimen seems difficult for people because we have been accustomed to eating a diet full of refined carbohydrates, processed foods, high proteins and high fats. These diets are very addictive and have been etched in our mind as a normal way of eating daily. In actuality, this way of eating should not be the norm but the caviar to be eaten occasionally, if at all. A diet full of fruits and vegetables should be the normal daily diet. Therefore a shift in mindset of what consists of healthy food choices needs to occur.

I believe in water fasting; however, most people cannot do water fasts. The incorporation of fruits and vegetables in this program and how it is structured helps detoxify and heal our bodies while reaping some of the benefits of water fasting. Most of the patients I see with chronic medical problems are advised to eat a healthy balanced diet along with exercise. I usually ask my patients to tell me what a typical day of eating is like for them. Most of their description of a typical daily diet includes lots of protein, fatty meals with refined carbohydrates, and minimal fruits and vegetables. The vegetables are usually cooked in oil or butter, and/or the fruits are sometimes dipped in caramel, chocolate, or whipped cream. This is not considered a healthy eating plan. Instead of their health improving, they are getting sicker requiring more and more medications.

Most of us love fruits. Eating fruit is strongly encouraged because eating fruit is easy to do. We want to focus on foods that are in their original state which can be found in nature. We want to avoid any fruits and vegetables that are not fresh. For example, any processed foods, fruits and/or vegetables that are cooked, frozen, or packaged should be avoided as much as possible. These foods have fortifying substances and/or preservatives in them that are not natural for the human body.

In our seven-day eating plan, there are separate *fruit days* and *vegetables days*. The fruit days consist of eating all types of fruits and drinking water the whole day. The regimen is to eat fruits and drink water on Mondays, Wednesdays, and Fridays in order to detoxify and heal the body. Tuesdays, Thursdays, Saturdays, and Sundays are our vegetable days. On these days we focus on eating whole-food plant based meals. We encourage that on our vegetable days we eat breakfast like a *king*, lunch like a *queen* and dinner like a *pauper*, especially if weight loss is the goal. I recommend that you stop eating your last meal at least 3 hours prior to going to sleep to prevent digestion problems. The seven day eating plan is then repeated weekly. Please refer to the tables below. *When you embark on this journey and you cannot do a full day of eating fruits, start with half a day of fruits and the other half, eat salads.* Gradually, do this until you can do a full day of fruits where you will reap the most benefits. Eat whole food plant based meals mostly on the other days.

On this plan, we also allow two meat meals a week. Our preferred meal plan is eating plant based meals. However, we understand that many people who start this journey are older in age and have been eating unhealthy foods for a long time. They come from eating the standard high fat, high carbohydrate, and high protein diet. They do not feel well and just want to feel better. Therefore, it is important to gradually introduce them to eating plant based meals as the main staple. In allowing two meat meals a week, they will get the health benefits of eating plant based foods, and still maintain some familiarity and control over what they are eating so they can be successful on the plan. Eventually, as they continue to see improved health benefits and wellness with eating wholesome plant based food, the goal would be that they will transition to eating plant based foods one hundred percent.

I strongly recommend eating a variety of fruits and vegetables on this program. Such foods are rich in flavonoids and fiber. The fiber in fruits and vegetables breaks down slowly, therefore slowing down metabolism and promoting satiety. Fruits and vegetables are healthy because they have the ability to lower cholesterol, manage blood pressure and improve gut health. They are low in calories and high in antioxidants, like polyphenols, which helps manage, control weight and reduce visceral fat. Visceral fat is the fat which surrounds abdominal organs and increases the risk of chronic diseases. There have been many people who have succeeded on this program, improved their chronic medical conditions and have minimized the use of medications. The transformation of weight loss, decrease in blood sugar numbers, and blood pressure numbers happens quickly. Therefore, we strongly recommend you partner with your healthcare Provider on this journey to guide you in adjusting your medications as you get the positive results.

Where do I get my Protein from on this program?

This is a question that is asked a lot? There are plenty of plant based foods that provide our body with enough protein. Eating a predominantly plant based diet is healthy for our body.

Animal protein is not the only source of protein. Plant protein is found in legumes (beans), vegetables and fruits. Plant protein is easier for our body to digest than animal protein and it does not require the energy it takes to digest animal protein. Plant protein does not become rotten like animal based protein when consumed, therefore we do not get the bad odor and constipation commonly associated with the elimination of animal foods.

Are you ready to take the challenge?

Whether you want to prevent, stabilize or reverse chronic conditions such as High blood Pressure, Diabetes Mellitus type II, High Cholesterol, Heart Disease and Obesity or simply shed some pounds, the Renew Health Transformation Program can help you make a change that will impact the rest of your life. You probably have heard and read many myths about carbohydrates and its effect on the body. I want you to forget all you have heard and try it for yourself to test the validity of the program.

The Renew Health Transformation Program works but like with everything worthwhile in life, it requires discipline, will-power, and consistency. The program will work for you if you work it. This is a healthy journey that when followed will help you for the rest of your life. I want you to succeed however, if you go off the eating plan, jump right on a *"fruit day"* to help you get back on track and detoxify your body. When this program is done right, you should lose *one* to *two* pounds on the scale the day after a *fruit* day. You have to be mindful on your vegetable days by not eating too much *salt* and/or fat. High sodium food will cause you to retain water which shows up on the scale as weight gain but it is your body actually holding on to water because of the salt. Ultimately as you continue with the program, you would lose fat and see visible results.

I highly recommend watching the videos on the YouTube channel: **Dr Owusu Skin Care & Wellness** for educational content, understanding, motivation and testimonials.

Below is a sample 7-day eating plan that can be repeated for 4 weeks and more. If you are unable to commit to the 28-Day challenge, try this life changing challenge for 7 days to reap the award-winning benefits. In addition to the plant-based foods, the program encourages the increased consumption of water, movement, rest and sunlight for total wellness. The Program cycle is for 28 days (4 weeks). The goal is that at the end of the 28 days, with the positive results obtained, we will learn how to make healthy food choices that can be incorporated into a long-term healthy lifestyle. The program can be utilized as a transitional lifestyle change for the maintenance of our health and well-being or can be implemented and repeated as often as needed.

Anyone can do this program without the supplements, however to maximize the benefits, it is strongly encouraged that you take advantage of the natural herb supplements that are recommended with the program.

These all-natural supplements are called: **Cell Support Formula** and **PowerFood Formula** which can be purchased at: **DrOwellness.com** or **buydro.com. The Cell Support Formula** (provides energy, improves cognitive function and curbs appetite) and the **PowerFood Formula** (strengthens overall health with essential nutrients, vitamins, and minerals).

Please follow an *option plan* below that best fits your needs and goals.

The 7-Day Eating Plan
(Repeat for 4 weeks or as long as you want)

Option One (For Health & Weight Loss Goals)

	Monday	Tuesday	Wednesday	Thursday	Friday	Saturday	Sunday
AM	Fruits	Starchy Carbohydrate Steamed Vegetables Salad + Fruit	Fruits	Starchy Carbohydrate Steamed Vegetables Salad + Fruit	Fruits	Starchy Carbohydrate Steamed Vegetables Salad + Fruit	Starchy Carbohydrate Steamed Vegetables Salad + Fruit
Snack	Fruits		Fruits		Fruits		
Afternoon	Fruits	Starchy Carbohydrate Steamed Vegetables Salad + Fruit	Fruits	Starchy Carbohydrate Steamed Vegetables Salad + Fruit	Fruits	Starchy Carbohydrate, Steamed Vegetables, Salad (or) Protein (4oz) & Veggies & Salad	Starchy Carbohydrate, Steamed Vegetables, Salad (or) Protein (4oz) & Veggies & Salad
Snack	Fruits		Fruits		Fruits		
PM	Fruits	Fruits & Vegetables	Fruits	Fruits & Vegetables	Fruits	Fruits & Vegetables	Fruits & Vegetables
Snack	Fruits		Fruits		Fruits		

The 7-Day Eating Plan
(Repeat for 4 weeks & or as long as you want)

Option Two (For Health Goal *but* No Weight Loss)

	Monday	Tuesday	Wednesday	Thursday	Friday	Saturday	Sunday
AM	Starchy Carbohydrate Steamed Vegetables Salad	Starchy Carbohydrate Steamed Vegetables Salad	Starchy Carbohydrate Steamed Vegetables Salad	Starchy Carbohydrate Steamed Vegetables Salad	Starchy Carbohydrate Steamed Vegetables Salad	Starchy Carbohydrate Steamed Vegetables Salad	Starchy Carbohydrate Steamed Vegetables Salad
Snack	Fruits	Fruits	Fruits	Fruits	Fruits	Fruits	Fruits
After-noon	Starchy Carbohydrate Steamed Vegetables Salad	Starchy Carbohydrate Steamed Vegetables Salad	Starchy Carbohydrate Steamed Vegetables Salad	Starchy Carbohydrate Steamed Vegetables Salad	Starchy Carbohydrate Steamed Vegetables Salad	Starchy Carbohydrate Steamed Vegetables Salad	Starchy Carbohydrate Steamed Vegetables Salad
Snack	Fruits	Fruits	Fruits	Fruits	Fruits	Fruits	Fruits
PM	Starchy Carbohydrate Steamed Vegetables Salad	Starchy Carbohydrate Steamed Vegetables Salad	Starchy Carbohydrate Steamed Vegetables Salad	Starchy Carbohydrate Steamed Vegetables Salad	Starchy Carbohydrate Steamed Vegetables Salad	Starchy Carbohydrate, Steamed Vegetables, Salad (or) Protein (4oz) & Veggies & Salad	Starchy Carbohydrate, Steamed Vegetables, Salad (or) Protein (4oz) & Veggies & Salad
Snack	Fruits	Fruits	Fruits	Fruits	Fruits	Fruits	Fruits

Examples of Starchy Carbohydrates (no oil)

White Potato, Sweet Potato, Rice (white or brown), Quinoa, Oatmeal, Beans, Corn, etc.

Boiled, raw, baked, broil or air-fry (best)-(no oil)

Vegetables

All Vegetables – boiled, raw, baked, broil or air-fry (no oil)

Fruits

All Fruits allowed

What can I Drink?

Water, Water, Water and more Water! *(If you are under a medical restriction for fluids, please follow your doctor's advice).*

Fresh fruit or vegetable infused water

Hot or Cold Herbal Tea with no sugar

Nuts

1 oz. nuts (2x a week)

Not on (M, W, F) - not on Fruit days (If weight loss is your goal, be mindful of nuts until you hit your goal weight).

Do Not Eat or Drink

No High Fat Meats (Fatty Red Meat. Chicken with skin, Sausage, Bacon)

No Dairy (Cheese & Milk)

No Oil

No Butter

No Fried Food

No White or Brown Sugar

No Soda, Diet Soda, Juices or other drinks

No Junk Food

No Processed Foods

No Alcohol

No Smoking

How about Exercise?

Walk at least 30 minutes a day (if you can) and/or

Resistance Training 2-3 times/week (if you can)

What are some Detox symptoms?

As your body starts healing, it is going to detox by getting rid of toxins. You can expect symptoms such as:

Headache

Diarrhea

Cold/Flu-like symptoms

Rash

Itching

Fatigue and/or more.

What are some benefits of this?

Better GI symptoms

Improvement in blood pressure

Improvement in diabetic numbers

Better quality sleep

Improvement in lung issues

Improvement in cholesterol

Improvement in pain level

Improvement in Autoimmune symptoms

Weight loss and much, much more.

Eating Out (Restaurants or Engagements)

When you are dining away from home, plan ahead the foods you can allow yourself to eat according to the plan. You can still follow the Renew Health Transformation Program to satisfaction. On the program you are allowed two protein meals a week. If eating a starchy carbohydrate meal during this time is difficult, then these are the perfect times to include your allowed meat meals.

Sample Meals at Restaurants

1. Lean Protein + cooked vegetables + Salad (or)

2. Starchy Carbohydrate (rice or potato) + Beans + cooked vegetables + salad

Fast Food Restaurants (*limited amount*)

Salad with no meat

Baked Potato with no topping (can top it vegetable chili and/or Salsa)

Bean Burrito

Vegetable Bowls

Vegetable Sandwiches

Impossible Whopper/King without cheese

Steamed Vegetables

Fruits

Maintenance

Once you reach your goal in your health journey, you can switch into "*maintenance*" mode. You can incorporate **one** to **two** fruit days a week or *none* to your health journey. Eat a low-fat plant based diet which includes starchy carbohydrates (with no oil), vegetables and fruits with a large salad daily.

Practice intuitive eating, stop eating when you are satisfied and full (not stuffed), and start eating when you are hungry. I highly recommend that you weigh yourself everyday as a practice to maintain your weight by analyzing how your body responds to the foods you eat and the condiments and seasoning you use.

If you start gaining weight, start back an all *fruit day* for detoxification. If you eat foods that are off the plan at any time (special occasions, holidays and/or vacations), go back to an all *fruit day* and follow the seven day eating plan until your body feels better again. Health and wellness is our portion. That is what God wants for us and we should want it for ourselves as well. We can heal our body, lose weight fast, and improve our spiritual, mental, and physical well-being. God wants us to be content, experience love, joy, peace, vitality, and wellness in our lives!

Focus Point.

Thank you for choosing the 28-Day Renew Health Transformation Program! Your decision will improve your health and increase your vitality and well-being! The effort you put in is the health benefit you will get back!

Congratulations Renew Health Warriors and God Bless You!!!

Chapter Ten

Testimonials

Patient A: TP (48 years old)
Started the Program: April 2022

Desired Goal: Weight Loss, Improvement in Gut Health & Management of Chronic Health Issues including Lupus and Eye Health.

Outcome: From April 2022 to July 2022 (4 months), TP achieved and exceeded her personal weight goal (lost 41.4 pounds) and noticed a decrease in her Lupus symptoms, eye pain and eye floaters secondary to retinal detachment. TP has made significant strides in relieving symptoms of constipation. Has overall improved vitality and wellness.

Patient B: LB (83 years old)
Started the Program: June 2022

Desired Goal: Improvement in General Well-being and better management of Diabetes Mellitus Type 2

Outcome: From June to August 2022, LB went from being on a scheduled insulin regimen (2 types of insulin 3 times a day) for Insulin Dependent Type 2 to diet controlled with sliding scale as needed. LB has lost 24 pounds and remains in pursuit of maximizing his weight management. He states he has more energy and feels better than he ever has.

Patient C: VB (77 years old)
Started the Program: June 2022

Desired Goal: Blood Pressure Management and Weight Loss

Outcome: Prior to starting the program VB was hypertensive and took 3 blood pressure medications. In one week, VB's blood pressure normalized. VB is no longer taking any blood pressure medications. VB's weight loss continues as well.

Patient D: MT (70 years old)
Started the Program: April 2022

Desired Goal: Blood Pressure and Diabetes Mellitus Type 2 management

Outcome: From April to July 2022, MT's blood pressure and diabetic numbers significantly improved resulting in no longer requiring blood pressure medications and diabetic medications. MT suffered from chronic constipation previously and now has improved gut regularity. MT has also seen an improvement in Hyperlipidemia, GERD and Heart Disease symptoms.

Patient E: MC (60 years old)
Started the Program: May 2022

Desired Goal: Pain management, Weight loss, and improvement in General Well-being.

Outcome: From May to July 2022, MC lost 35 pounds and remains in pursuit of maximizing weight management. MC no longer suffers from generalized joint pain, and has seen improvement in Cognitive and Thyroid Function.

Patient F: AO (20 years old)
Started Program: June 2022

Desired Goal: Improvement in Hyperthyroidism symptoms

Outcome: From June 2022 to July 2022, AO's symptoms of Hyperthyroidism, such as palpitation, elevated heart rate, hand and voice tremors, eye bulging, and thyroid gland enlargement (goiter), improved with diet. AO did not require medications for Hyperthyroidism. As a benefit, AO also noticed an improvement in Pre-menstrual symptoms (PMS).

Patient G: SP (65 years old)
Started Program: May 2022

Desired Goal: Weight Loss and Improvement in Respiratory Status

Outcome: From May 2022 to August 2022, SP has lost over 40 pounds. SP was dependent on steroids because of poor respiratory status which has improved with the program.

These are just a few of the testimonials we receive regularly. Visit our website *(renewhealth2.com or DrOwellness.com)* or our YouTube channel (*Dr. Owusu Skincare & Wellness*) to see some more testimonials.

Chapter Eleven

Sample Recipes

Low-Fat Plant Food Recipes

Tomato Blend

- 3 Roma Tomatoes
- ¼ Small Onion
- 1 Jalapeño or Green Pepper
- ½ teaspoon salt

Blend all ingredients together and refrigerate for use

Curry Vegetable Stir Fry

- 1 Green Bell Pepper
- I red Bell Pepper
- 1 Large Onion
- 2 cups Broccoli florets
- ¼ cup of Oatmeal or a mall potato
- I tablespoon of yellow curry
- 1 teaspoon of Adobe
- 1 tablespoon of Garlic powder
- I tablespoon of Onion powder

Directions: Cut all vegetables into big stir fry sizes.

Place ¼ cup of water in a cooking pot, Add the Green pepper, red pepper and onions and cover and let cook for 5 minutes.

Place the Oatmeal in a blender with 1 cup of water, add the curry, garlic powder, onion powder, and adobe and blend, pour the blend in the pot with vegetables, stir fry together, cook and let it cook for 10 minutes.

Bean Stew

- 1 can of Beans of choice
- 1 can of petite tomatoes
- 1 Medium onion chopped
- 1 tablespoon of Garlic Powder
- 1 tablespoon of Onion Powder
- 1 teaspoon of Adobe

Directions: Place a cooking bowl on medium heat, add ¼ cup of water and sauté onions. Add tomatoes, garlic powder, onion powder and seasoning, and beans, mix and cover to cook for 10 minutes on low heat.

Pico de Gallo

- 6 Roma Tomatoes (diced)
- 1 Medium-Large Onion (minced)
- 2 Jalapeno pepper, seeded and minced; or Green Pepper

- 3-4 tablespoons chopped fresh Cilantro
- (2) Fresh Lime, juiced
- Salt (1/2 teaspoon) and ground pepper to take (1/2 teaspoon)

Directions: Mix all ingredients together and refrigerator

Curry Vegetable Stir Fry

- 1 Green Bell Pepper
- I red Bell Pepper
- 1 Large Onion
- 2 cups Broccoli florets
- ¼ cup of Oatmeal or a mall potato
- I tablespoon of yellow curry
- 1 teaspoon of Adobe
- 1 tablespoon of Garlic powder
- I tablespoon of Onion powder

Directions: Cut all vegetables into big stir fry sizes.

Place ¼ cup of water in a cooking pot, Add the Green pepper, red pepper and onions and cover and let cook for 5 minutes.

Place the Oatmeal in a blender with 1 cup of water, add the curry, garlic powder, onion powder, and adobe and blend, pour the blend in the pot with vegetables, stir fry together, cook and let it cook for 10 minutes.

Bean Stew

- 2 cans of Beans of choice
- 1 can of petite tomatoes
- 1 Medium onion chopped
- 1 tablespoon of Garlic Powder
- 1 tablespoon of Onion Powder
- 1 teaspoon of Adobe

Directions: Place a cooking bowl on medium heat, add ¼ cup of water and sauté onions. Add tomatoes, garlic powder, onion powder and seasoning, beans, mix and cover to cook for 10 minutes on low-medium heat.

Vegetable Stir-Fry with Peanut Sauce

- 2 cups of Frozen mixed vegetables or (vegetables of choice)
- 2 cups of Frozen cut okra (un-breaded) or (vegetables of choice)
- 2 Medium to large Onion (minced)
- 1 tablespoon of tomato paste
- 2 tablespoons PB Fit peanut butter
- 1 + 1/4 cup of water
- Seasoning of choice

Directions: Place cooking pot on heat, place 1/4 water, add onions and stir fry. Mix 2 tablespoons of PB Fit peanut butter in 1 cup of water and mix, then add mixture in cooking onion mixture. Add to the mixture the tomato paste and stir. Add the vegetables, 1 cup of water, seasoning, stir and cover to cook for 10 minutes.

Serve over rice, potatoes or eat by itself.

Vegetable Bean Salad

- 1 can Beans of choice
- 1 can Corn (drained)
- 1 can of Sweet Peas (drained)
- 2 tablespoon Maple Syrup
- 2 tablespoons of Dijon Mustard

Directions: Combine all ingredients and mix together.

Serve over rice, potato, sweet potato, and with green vegetables.

Pasta Sauce (Oil Free)

- 12 oz. Tomato Paste
- 3 cups Water
- 1/4 cup Sundried Tomatoes (oil-free)
- 1 tablespoon Italian Seasoning
- 1 teaspoon Garlic powder
- 1 teaspoon Onion powder
- 1/4 teaspoon crushed red pepper flakes
- 2 tablespoon Maple Syrup

Directions: Blend all ingredients together. Once blended, cook the sauce on the stove in a pot, cover for 30 minutes (stir occasionally) or cook it in Instant Pot or pressure cooker x 10 minutes.

Baked Vegetables

(Brussel Sprouts; or Broccoli; or California Medley; or Asparagus, etc.)

Wash Fresh Vegetables; wipe off excess water; season with garlic powder, onion powder, Adobo, Mrs. Dash or seasoning of choice. Place vegetables in a baking dish, spray top with PAM spray, cover with foil and bake in the oven at 375 degrees for 45 minutes or until tender.

Air-Fry French Fries or Sweet Potato Fries

Cut up 1-2 white potatoes or sweet potatoes, season to taste, place in an air-fryer and cook for 15 to 20 minutes until tender and crunchy. Serve with catsup, mustard and/or Sriracha hot sauce and Vegetables.

"The Effort you put in
is the Health Result or Benefit you will get back"

This is not the End but the Beginning!

About the Author

Dr. Jacqueline Owusu (Dr. JackieO) is a physician, author, Christain motivational speaker, entrepreneur, creator and founder of a skincare line and mother of two boys. She is actively pursuing her call to motivate, encourage and educate others to live a burden free life by promoting a healthy lifestyle in order for others to achieve wellness in their spirit, soul and body.

Dr. Owusu was born in Ghana, West Africa and came to the United States in 1981 to join her family. She attended Elementary school and High School in New York City. After high school, Dr. Owusu received an undergraduate degree in Biochemistry and a Masters Degree in Public Administration (MPA). She went on to pursue a career in medicine by attending medical school where she was awarded a Doctor of Medicine degree (MD), specializing and becoming Board Certified in Internal Medicine.

As a practicing physician, Dr. Owusu felt a need to do more for her patients and herself. Patients were not being cured of their diseases and were requiring more and more medications without improvement. This prompted Dr. Owusu to seek answers. With prayer and guidance from God and educating herself in how to use nutrition and herbs to naturally heal the body, Dr. Owusu embarked on a healing journey for herself which has expanded to include the healing of others. This journey is what prompted the writing of this book as well as the 28-Day Renew Health Transformation Program and Coaching.

Dr. Owusu's other books in print are: *Forgive Yourself: For Your Father God has Forgiven You. Recognize & Appreciate The Little Miracles. Inspirational Steps to.* The books can be purchased on these websites **www.DrOwellness.com** or **www.buydro.com.**

For speaking engagement and inquiries, please contact Dr. Jacqueline Owusu at

talkwithdrj@gmail.com.

RENEW HEALTH CHALLENGE

Are you ready for the Challenge that can

Change and Impact the Rest of Your Life!

Visit…

renewyourhealthchallenge.com

Made in the USA
Columbia, SC
17 March 2023

13760271R00059